Apple Cider Vinegar

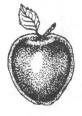

For Weight Loss & Good Health

Cynthia Holzapfel

Healthy Living Publications
Summertown, Tennessee

Cover design: Cynthia Holzapfel
Photography: Warren Jefferson

Published in the United States by
Healthy Living Publications
P.O. Box 99
Summertown, TN 38483
1-888-260-8458
www.bookpubco.com

Printed in the United States

ISBN 1-57067-127-3

07 06 05   4 5 6 7 8 9

Holzapfel, Cynthia, 1948-
  Apple cider vinegar for weight loss & good health / by Cynthia Holzapfel.
      p. cm.
Includes index.
  ISBN 1-57067-127-3
  1. Cider vinegar--Therapeutic use--Popular works. 2. Weight loss. I. Title.
  RM666.V55 H65 2002
  615'.321--dc21   2001007578

Apple Cider Vinegar for Weight Loss & Good Health is intended solely for informational and educational purposes and not as medical counseling. Please consult a medical or health professional if you have questions about any conditions related to your health. The publisher and author are not responsible for any adverse effects or consequences resulting from the use of any of the suggestions or preparations discussed in this book.

Table of Contents

Dedication

To the people of Orleans County, New York, for their support of apple farming through many generations of growers and canners,

And to my mother, who has never been afraid to consider new ideas and whose interest in learning has always been an inspiration.

Introduction

I grew up in apple country. Even the names in our area echoed that fact: Orchard Creek, the Apple Grove Inn. Western New York is one of the country's great apple growing areas, and I remember autumns where the bounty of apples was everywhere. In the little town where I lived, the storage lot in front of the local applesauce and vinegar plant sported giant pyramids of apples: red, yellow, and mixed colors. My friends and I would ride our horses through neighboring apple orchards, the idyllic setting for many hours of imaginary play. And there's not much that can beat the tangy crunch of a New York red delicious moments after it's picked from the tree.

Very little was discussed in my family about the healing or nutritive properties of apples, apart from the fact that my mother could make a great apple pie. The one thing that does stick in my memory is her use of apple cider vinegar and black tea bags on a particularly bad sunburn I got as a teenager. She was a thoroughly modern woman and a registered nurse to boot, but she understood how the application of a little home medicine could be as effective as anything on the pharmacy shelf.

We live in an amazing age of medical miracles where longevity continues to increase, and many of the threatening diseases which cut life short before 1900 have been seriously challenged by antibiotics. However, in the last twenty or thirty years, there has been a growing recognition of the limits of modern medicine to combat chronic illness. This awareness has lead many people to re-examine the healing potential of traditional, or "folk," medicine. These ancient restorative practices have their limitations and cannot compete with modern surgical practice or microbiology in the healing of traumatic injury or protecting against infectious disease. Still, folk medicine has its own strengths, arising from our intuitive understanding of the delicate interplay among the body's natural defense mechanisms. Folk medicine credits the role of the mind in the healing process and uses a variety of substances found in nature. Modern medical scientists are obsessed with isolating and identifying which specific chemical element of a substance may be crucial for a successful therapy. By contrast, natural healers are more inclined to use whole substances in as natural a form as possible. These healers have a firm belief that each element in a natural substance plays an interactive role which may never be understood. They appreciate that trying to separate these elements may only result in ineffective parts—the sum of which is much less than the whole.

Which brings us back to apples, the source of such wise sayings as "an apple a day keeps the doctor away." In the following pages I'll touch on how apples are transformed into the powerhouse of healing: apple cider vinegar. You'll learn how apple cider vinegar can be effective for weight loss and a handy tool in your medicine cabinet. My hope is that you'll find the information helpful in using this delicious gift of nature to increase the health and well being of you and your family.

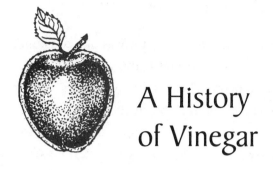

A History
of Vinegar

We have no idea when man began eating fermented foods. At some time in human history, we evolved from eating only fresh meat, fruits, grains, and vegetables, to including delicacies a little past their prime but still tasty and tempting. We're not the only species that has a fascination with "second generation" foods which are transformed by the action of bacteria and other single-celled organisms. Some birds, for instance, have been known to make fools of themselves after eating from a patch of fermented berries.

Vinegar through the ages

There is justified speculation that the use of vinegar parallels the advent of wine-making about 10,000 years ago. Around the world, wine is invariably the most popular fermented liquid (with beer running a close second). Although many fermented foods have been used to make a variety of vinegars, wine was most likely the first candidate. The use of vinegar by the Babylonians dates back to around 5000 BCE. The Babylonians creatively transformed not only the fruit of the date palm into wine and vinegar, but possibly the sap (which they might have harvested much like New Englanders tap maple trees for syrup). This sap may have been such a perfect medium for the bacteria that create vinegar, if the wine made from it was not consumed fairly quickly, vinegar would have been the inevitable and immediate result. It must have been delicious, because a large industry evolved in Babylonia for the mass production of vinegar.

Similarly, the use of vinegar in China appears in texts that date back to 1200 BCE. We know that wine was a part of Chinese culinary culture and that sour seasoning existed at that time; it's not much of a leap to imagine that the Chinese let wine sour to make a vinegar used to flavor foods. By 300 BCE, there is mention of sour sauces and salads which could have only been concocted using vinegar. The Chinese were also adept at using vinegar to preserve foods, not only to keep them for future use, but to transform them into new and delicious delicacies such as pickles. Although we can imagine that vinegar was an important staple in many cultures, the Chinese codified this importance through the writings of Wu Tzu-Mu in the Sung dynasty of 960-1279 AD, who stated, "the things that people cannot do without every day are firewood, rice, oil, salt, soybean sauce, tea, and vinegar."

Perhaps the most famous story of vinegar in history tells of a wager made between Queen Cleopatra of Egypt and Mark Anthony, a Roman general. Cleopatra bet that she could provide a feast for the two of them that would cost an unheard of sum. After the meal, Mark Anthony scoffed that there was no way their meal could have met the stipulations of the wager. Cleopatra requested a vial of vinegar be brought to her, at which point she removed a priceless pearl she was wearing and dropped it into the liquid. The pearl dissolved and Cleopatra drank the vinegar, thus winning the bet. To test this legend, renown vinegar historian and enthusiast Lawrence Diggs actually dissolved a cultured pearl in vinegar and published pictures of the process which you can see in his book, *Vinegar* (Authors Choice Press: Lincoln, Nebraska).

Medical and other applications

Hippocrates, the venerated Greek healer and father of modern medicine, recommended the use of vinegar (especially when combined with honey) in a variety of preparations to treat everything from coughs to bacterial infections. Vinegar is mentioned throughout the Bible both as a food and drink. Perhaps the most significant reference is to the Roman soldiers who offered Jesus a sponge soaked in vinegar to quench his thirst. Although this might seem an unusual offering, it helps to know that diluted vinegar (called *posca*) was a common beverage of poor Romans and Roman soldiers.

Another famous application of vinegar in history was used by the Carthagian general Hannibal as he attempted to cross the Alps—on elephants, no less. You can imagine the amount of room needed to move an elephant through these mountain passes, but Hannibal met this challenge in a creative fashion. He had the good fortune to be blocked by rocks whose chemical composition would be affected by vinegar, so he had the rocks heated, then split and crumbled by pouring vinegar over them.

The cuisine of the Middle Ages in Europe was marked by its lack of variety, but vinegar played an active role in providing some interest to the few foods available. It was often flavored with fruits and herbs. Many of the references to vinegar from this period in history tell about its use in preventing disease. Hildegard von Bingen, an 11th century healer, wrote of many uses of vinegar for cleansing the body and aiding digestion.

Vinegar was used in times of pestilence as an effective disinfectant. In what may be one of the first great urban legends, it was popularly reported that a small band of men were arrested for robbing the homes of unfortunate victims of the plague. The robbers claimed they were able to survive being in such close proximity to this highly infectious and virulent disease by covering themselves liberally with a combination of white wine vinegar, herbs, and camphor. The men also claimed they were able to protect themselves from inhaling any germs by daubing their noses with this concoction. They carried extra vials of it with them so they could regularly breathe its vapors and proceed without harm.

The history of the apple in America

Although apples as we know them today are not indigenous to the Americas, they are now such an integral part of our culture that we think of ourselves as "American as apple pie." Before European settlement, only a relative of flavorful apples, the crab apple, grew in North America. Beacon Hill in Boston is reputed to have been the site of the first American apple orchard, planted in 1625. George Washington and Thomas Jefferson were not only important American political leaders, they were notable agrarians and apple growers, as well.

One legendary American pioneer, John Chapman, became a fixture in history due to his relationship with the apple. From Leominster, Massachusetts, west of Boston, "Johnny Appleseed" traveled through New York to Ohio, Indiana, and Illinois sharing apple seeds and seedlings with frontier settlers. And in Ontario, Canada, John McIntosh discovered a variety of apple in 1796 whose name would have significance in the field of computers: the McIntosh apple.

Apple cider in colonial America

Apple cider was a popular beverage in the colonies, as it was in England at the time of the American Revolution. The Normans brought their taste for cider with them during their conquest of England, and the wine embargoes of the Hundred Years' War slowed the flow of French wine into England to a trickle, increasing the consumption of cider.

Although beer-making was popular in Northern Europe, it was cheaper to press apples for cider than it was to cook malt for beer, and by the mid-1600s, the brewing of cider had attained the same status in England as wine-making had in France. The bittersweet and bittersharp apples which were so favored for cider-making grew easily in the temperate English climate. At the pinnacle of cider's popularity, British horticulturalist John Worlidge cataloged every known cider apple of that time in his *A Treatise of Cider*. Even Capt. James Cook took cider with him on his voyages through the South Seas to help prevent scurvy among his crew.

Brewed beverages were also a safe bet in Europe before the advent of clean municipal drinking water, as lakes and rivers were common dumping grounds for raw sewage. Although drinking water in the American colonies was some of the best in the world, early Americans continued the practice of using alcoholic hard cider as a primary beverage. By the late 1800s, cider's importance began to wane, influenced by a growing American temperance movement among settlers of English descent and by German and Irish immigrants who preferred beer. However, apple cider vinegar had been firmly established as a staple in the medicine chests of folk practitioners and on the tables of American homemakers.

Apple cider vinegar in natural health care

I'd like to note the work of several well-known promoters of apple cider vinegar in recent years. In the early '50s a Vermont country doctor by the name of D.C. Jarvis published a small book on his observations of the use of apple cider vinegar by his rural patients to successfully treat a number of common ailments. *Folk Medicine* began as a way to organize these findings in a form he could leave to his daughter and grandchildren, but it evolved into one of the most popular treatises on the use of apple cider vinegar to promote health.

On many occasions Dr. Jarvis involved his patients in simple experiments to test whether taking apple cider vinegar would positively affect health. By analyzing urine samples he was able to detect patterns of changing acidity and alkalinity in the body as a response to illness. He observed that the urine of patients who drank apple cider vinegar to combat the onset of acute illness (colds, flu, etc.) would return quickly to its normal acidity. Dr. Jarvis also made observations about regular use of apple cider vinegar to combat chronic conditions, such as high blood pressure, arthritis, and overweight. To prove that the success of these treatments was not the result of a placebo effect influenced by the faith of his patients, Dr. Jarvis also tested the use of apple cider vinegar on ailing farm animals and got similar positive results.

Paul C. Bragg, a pioneer of the mid-twentieth century health food movement, was a modern-day American promoter of a raw foods diet (as well as the use of fresh juices, untreated water, and vigorous exercise) for improving and maintaining health. He was also a strong advocate of the use of apple cider vinegar, especially with honey, as a healing beverage. Bragg's family made their own apple cider vinegar from the apples they grew and used it as a staple in their diet. His father drank a combination of cider vinegar and honey to relieve the fatigue of long hours working on a farm. While recovering from tuberculosis as a teenager, Bragg rediscovered this healthful elixir and credited his renewed vigor and strength to it. He went on to publish a number of books on apple cider vinegar, fasting, raw foods, and other subjects relating to health, diet, and fitness with his daughter Patricia Bragg.

Like Dr. Jarvis, Bragg believed the potassium and enzymes in apple cider vinegar (especially those found in organic, unfiltered cider vinegar) were the reasons for its effectiveness in promoting good health.

Apple cider vinegar for today's lifestyles

With the renewed interest in finding health solutions in our everyday diet, apple cider vinegar is back in the spotlight, along with soy, oats, blueberries, sea vegetables, and flaxseed, as one of a number of nutrient "power foods." It's part of a medically supported trend away from the overconsumption of commercially processed, packaged products in favor of eating more natural, whole foods.

Apple cider vinegar fits in well with the move many people are making toward more healthful, simple lifestyles. It is readily available, inexpensive, and extremely versatile. A dash of apple cider vinegar can be enough to liven up a plate of steamed vegetables, spike a salad, or give just the right amount of flavor to a sauce or dip. A simple tonic of vinegar, water, and honey can help maintain optimum body functioning or reduce weight. And, of course, there are many uses of apple cider vinegar as a handy tool in your medicine chest.

In order to understand why apple cider vinegar is so effective, we'll explore how it is made, then investigate the ways you can use it to lose weight and maintain good health.

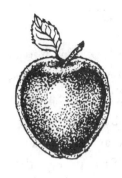

Apple Cider Vinegar: What it is and How to Make it

How juice turns to vinegar

Along with cheese, yogurt, wine, and beer, vinegar is one of many favorite foods which are created by bacteria and yeasts. Most vinegar begins as fruit juice which is exposed first to yeasts, then bacteria, which work on fruit sugars in different ways. Initially these sugars are fermented by yeast to create alcohol. Then specific bacteria break down the alcohol to form acetic acid, the main component in vinegar. Both the yeasts and bacteria that make vinegar are plentiful in nature, so after juices are extracted from fruits, these liquids naturally progress through stages of fermentation, then acetification. Vinegar is the result. The natural tendency of fruit juice to ferment explains why alcoholic beverages and vinegar have been staples in the diets of almost every culture around the world since before recorded history. In fact, the word vinegar comes from the French term "vin aigre," or sour wine. Vinegar can be made from any fruit, many grains (such as rice wine vinegar popular in Asian cuisine), and even wood chips. In the case of grains and wood, the starches in these substances are first converted to sugars so the fermentation process can begin.

If you've ever seen homemade vinegar, or perhaps had a bottle of wine that has "vinegared," you may have seen a thick, filmy substance floating in it, often near the top. This fibrous substance is called "mother of vinegar." It consists of cellulose that results from the interaction of the bacteria with the alcohol. Sometimes mother of vinegar is thought to be responsible for the creation of vinegar, much the same way as yogurt starter makes more yogurt, but it is more a result of the process than the initiator. A family of bacteria called acetobacters are actually responsible for the conversion of alcohol into vinegar.

Acetobacters are plentiful in our natural environment and require oxygen in order to survive and grow. If alcoholic beverages like apple cider are exposed to the open air for a period of time, the interaction of the acetobacters and oxygen in the air facilitates the conversion of the alcohol into vinegar. Because the mother of vinegar is likely to have a concentration of acetobacters clinging to it, it can be used to introduce these organisms into cider. The nature of these bacteria is somewhat mysterious, and even modern scientists disagree as to how many kinds of acetobacters actually exist. This makes the isolation of a pure strain of bacteria for vinegar-making as much an art as a science.

As cider is transformed into vinegar, the alcoholic content drops and the acidity rises. The simplest way to tell whether the process is complete is by tasting it; no odor or flavor of alcohol should be present. The strength of the vinegar is determined by the amount of alcohol in the cider. Since much of the vinegar for household use is around 4 to 6 percent acidity, the alcohol content of the cider needs to be about that percentage as well.

Making apple cider vinegar

If you'd like to make your own vinegar from cider, fill a sterilized wide-mouthed jar about two-thirds with hard apple cider.

Add to the cider either a little unpasteurized, unfiltered organic apple cider vinegar or some mother of vinegar (available at some health food stores or where brewing ingredients are sold). Cover the top with cheesecloth, so the vinegar bacteria will have access to oxygen without being contaminated by insects. Set the jar for about 4 weeks in any dark place that stays around room temperature. The best indicator of when the vinegar is ready is by taste, the only method that was employed for centuries. When the vinegar is ready, there should be no more flavor of alcohol. If you have a wine-testing kit, you can test the vinegar until it is about 5 or 6 percent acidity. (For anyone who is intrigued by the idea of making their own vinegar, Lawrence Diggs' *Vinegar* is a great comprehensive guide for the amateur vinegar enthusiast.)

This simple household method was most likely the first way vinegar was produced. As the use of vinegar became more popular and there was more demand for commercial production, manufacturers developed a process using wooden barrels laid on their sides and filled halfway with wine. This technique is often known as the field process or Orleans method (for the French town where this method was most notably employed). With the barrels on their sides, rather than upright, more surface area of the wine was exposed to the air. To facilitate this exposure, holes were usually drilled at either end of the barrels and covered with fine mesh screen to keep out contaminants. To shorten the time needed for fermentation, other methods were developed where wine or cider was passed through a tank filled with wood chips, charcoal, or even corn cobs to increase the surface area that came in contact with the air.

During fermentation (especially during commercial production where great quantities of quality vinegar are made), it's important not to disturb the vinegar in progress. If the mother of vinegar which normally floats on the surface is moved, it may sink to the bottom of the container and decompose, adversely affecting the flavor and quality of the vinegar. The famous French scientist Louis Pasteur, who wrote numerous articles on the bacteriological processes involved in making vinegar, was instrumental in inventing a type of wooden "raft" that would float at the top of vinegar barrels and help keep the mother on top of the vinegar. Time is also an important factor in making truly flavorful vinegar, much the same way as aging makes great cheese or wine.

Apple cider vinegar nutrition

Although most commercial vinegar these days is filtered to remove the mother and any sediments, it is often these elements that give vinegar its character and healthful qualities. Sadly, many people feel a clear vinegar is a superior product because it's more aesthetically appealing, so producers comply by filtering and pasteurizing the vinegar they make. This process stops the activity of the acetobacter bacteria. The result is vinegar whose quality can be regulated and assured, but is lacking some of the vital qualities that makes it so effective for good health. Removing the sediments and mother of vinegar also reduces the complexity of flavors in the vinegar. Like refined flour and pasteurized juices that have had nutrients removed or destroyed, vinegar that is filtered and pasteurized may be commercially acceptable, but less effective nutritionally. The quality vinegar that Dr. Jarvis and the Braggs were so enthusiastic about contained all the health-promoting qualities of the apples from which it was made.

Apples are nutritional powerhouses and truly deserving of the legendary phrase: "An apple a day keeps the doctor away." They contain a wide range of nutrients, such as pectin (soluble fiber), beta-carotene (an antioxidant), and a number of minerals. The most plentiful mineral is potassium; one apple contains almost 10% of all the potassium you need daily.

Just take a look at the list of nutrients below to see the potential in apples and apple cider vinegar.

I MEDIUM APPLE (138 g)

81 calories	.1 mg niacin
115.8 g water	.08 mg pantothenic
.3 g protein	1 mg sodium
21.1 g carbohydrates	10 mg calcium
.5 g fat	6 mg magnesium
2.8 g dietary fiber	.05 mg zinc
74 IU A	.062 mg manganese
8 mg C	159 mg potassium
.02 mg B_2	10 mg phosphorus
.07mg B_6	.25 mg iron
4 mcg folic acid	.057 mg copper
.02 mg B_1	

CIDER VINEGAR
(1 Tablespoon = 15 g)

2 calories	1 mg calcium
14.1 g water	1 mg phosphorus
15 mg potassium	.1 mg iron

From *Food Values of Portions Commonly Used, 15th ed.*, Jean A. T. Pennington (HarperCollins, New York)

There's an advantage to drinking some apple cider vinegar each day that you wouldn't get just by eating raw apples. The fermentation process that creates hard apple cider, then sours the cider to make vinegar, adds important enzymes and acids to the original apples. Many people feel that these elements are important to the processes of healing and weight loss. In the chapters that follow, we'll explore the role that all the nutrients in apple cider vinegar play in increasing your health and vitality.

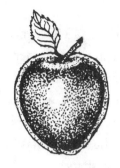

Losing Weight with Apple Cider Vinegar

Can apple cider vinegar really help you lose weight? I believe it can. In order to convince you, let me explain a little bit about fat, the role it plays in our bodies, and how our bodies work naturally to process and eliminate it. If you understand some of these nutrition basics, it will be easy to see how apple cider vinegar can be the basis of a successful weight loss strategy.

What does fat do for our bodies?

Fat plays a crucial role in keeping us healthy, so even if we're watching our waistlines, we have to have a certain amount of the right kind of fat in our diet. Perhaps the most important thing fat does for us is provide a storehouse of fuel we can draw on for our daily activities. We can burn protein for fuel if we need to, and carbohydrates give us instant energy, but it's fat that provides the resources to keep us going over the long haul.

Besides being an energy source, fat insulates our bodies and keeps them warm. Have you ever noticed how your appetite increases as the amount of daylight decreases with the coming of winter? The temptation posed by Christmas cookies doesn't come just from your sweet tooth. There's a biological imperative driving the urge to add to your fat stores and create an extra layer of protection for the winter ahead. As an added bonus, this extra protection will provide a safety net against starvation should your food supply run short over the winter. (This is not necessarily something we have to worry about in these modern times, but our bodies have not evolved over the course of human history as quickly as our ability to ensure that we have enough to eat.) The shape and size of this protective layer is determined by heredity and our sex, much to the consternation of many women who are concerned about their shapes.

You might not be aware of the fat in your body that's way below the surface, but fats are an integral component of all our cells and provide a cushion for our hearts, lungs, livers, and other organs. Fats are involved in the reaction of certain enzymes and the activity of some hormones, as well as beta-carotene and vitamins A, D, E, and K. All of these vitamins need the presence of fat in order to be absorbed by the body.

Finally, fats are also responsible for the health of your nervous system. When they combine with the mineral phosphorus, they create a substance called lecithin. Lecithin plays an important role in creating neurotransmitters, the chemicals that work in your brain to regulate your mood, appetite, and cognitive functions (your ability to learn, remember, etc.).

Most of the fats you consume are separated from the food you eat during the digestive process and recombined in various ways so your body can use them. However, some of the fats your body needs can't be processed from other nutrients and must be obtained through your diet. These essential fatty acids—omega-6 and omega-3—work in opposition to each other. Omega-6s increase blood pressure, blood clotting, and cell proliferation. (You could think of these as "active" responses.) Omega-3 fatty acids evoke exactly the opposite, more calming responses. It's the balance of these two functions that brings about a positive state of health. Omega-6 and omega-3 fatty acids are found in a variety of foods: flaxseed oil, canola and other vegetable oils, walnuts, wheat germ, and dark green leafy vegetables, as well as fish and other seafood, to name just a few.

Science has made great strides in the last 30 years in identifying the health problems caused by eating animal fats. Most of the fat in meat, fish, and dairy products is saturated fat. The more saturated fat you eat, the more likely it is that your cholesterol level will rise, thereby raising your chances for heart disease and stroke. An exception to this rule applies to the saturated fats from plant sources: coconut, avocado, and palm oil. Nutritional researchers are now questioning whether these fats should carry the same stigma as those from animal sources. Even though they are saturated, these "tropical" oils have a different chemical composition than animal fats and do not clog arteries or cause heart disease. By getting more fats from vegetable sources such as olive oil, canola oil, and fresh nuts and seeds, you can reduce your chances for heart disease, some cancers, high cholesterol, inflammation, arthritis, and other health problems.

There are many ways in which apple cider vinegar helps us to make the best use of the fats we consume in order to improve health and promote weight loss. First let's look at the ways fat works in the body, for better and for worse.

How does fat make us fat?

The way most of us get fat is by eating more food than we need for our daily bodily functions. Much has been said lately about the success of low-fat diets. Although it's easy for your body to convert the fats you eat to fat on your hips, the truth is you cannot eliminate fat from your diet, then binge on pasta and bread and expect to stay slim. If you eat more calories than you burn, the pounds will eventually add up.

There are many factors that can either act alone, or in combination, to contribute to being overweight. In his book *Staying Healthy with Nutrition*, Dr. Elson Haas offers a list of theories and causes:

General	Specific
Metabolic rate	Excess calories and/or fats
Set point	Excess sugar refined foods
Fat cell type and number	Overeating
	Slow liver metabolism
Family Influences	Nutrient deficiencies
Heredity	Low thyroid function
Eating patterns	Lack of exercise
Food choices	Food allergies
Family relationship	Yeast infections
Food as security substitute	Parasites
Psychological attitudes	Insulin insensitivity
Self-image within family	Emotional factors
	Fat body self-image

If your weight is average for your height and body type, it's more than likely that you'll have a set number of fat cells throughout your adult years. When you gain or lose weight, these fat cells don't multiply; they either expand or shrink depending on the amount of fat they have to accommodate. You increase the number of fat cells you have when you grow as an infant and again as a teenager, and if you overeat during these stages of life, you increase your chances of making more fat cells than you would otherwise. Sometimes these cells are so full of fat already that the body is triggered to make more of them.

You can't make a fat cell go away naturally. This is why liposuction and other fat-removing surgeries have become so popular in recent years. And if it wasn't bad enough that you cannot diet your fat cells away, it turns out these cells have a powerful drive to survive. Shrinking your fat cells triggers a strong message to your brain to eat more, creating a huge challenge to your will to diet.

Carrying extra pounds increases your chances for disease and chronic health problems, such as cancer (especially of the breast, colon, stomach, gallbladder, and prostate), heart disease, diabetes, kidney disease, stroke, arthritis, varicose veins, and infertility. Clearly, being in good shape has a marked effect on your quality of life and longevity.

How does the body process and eliminate fat?

As shown in Dr. Hass' list on page 24, there are several mechanisms that work to keep the body slim. Metabolism, the overall activity of the body, is one of the most important of these. It is affected by our age, sex, diet, the amount of activity we get, how well our thyroid functions, how much sleep we get, how much body fat we have, our body temperature, our weight, and our genetic make-up.

It's a well-known fact that people with muscles burn fat, and the more muscles they have, the more fat they'll burn. Unfit people tend to burn more carbohydrates than fat, because their short-term energy needs can be amply met by what they eat in their daily diet. It is only during long stretches of activity that your body turns to your fat stores for energy.

Another theory of how your body uses energy and burns fat relates to the concept of a "set point." Your set point determines what level of activity will trigger the urge to eat and influences how much you want to eat. It's a natural "cruise control" mechanism that some nutrition researchers think is regulated by your fat cells. We've seen how fat cells don't like to be too thin. How comfortable these cells are with their size will determine your set point and whether your metabolism will kick in quickly or languish in the doldrums.

Your set point is also established by how sensitive your cells have become to insulin. Glucose is the simple sugar that results from the breakdown of many of the foods we eat. When the level of glucose in your blood increases, your pancreas secretes more insulin to move that glucose to the cells. If your blood sugar is at a consistently high level, your cells will be constantly exposed to insulin and may develop a condition known as insulin insensitivity, one of the main causes of diabetes in adults. As the cells become less receptive to the activity of insulin, glucose remains in the bloodstream and your body thinks it has all the energy it can use—and then some. In this condition, it won't get any signals to burn fat.

Along with a set point, there is a tendency for some people to create more body heat when they eat than other people. This process is called thermogenesis. Imagine two furnaces; one is tightly built and properly drafted, and the other has a chimney that doesn't draw well. If you burn the same type and amount of wood in both furnaces, you'll get a roaring fire and lots of heat from the first furnace. The fire in the poorly drafted furnace never seems to take off. The same thing can happen to people with different metabolisms. Lower thermogenesis can also be caused by insulin insensitivity. When the cells aren't taking up much blood sugar, the amount of heat they produce is also low.

Diets that are high in fats and refined carbohydrates drive the body's blood sugar regulating mechanisms out of balance, resulting in insulin insensitivity and diabetes. Obesity and diabetes feed on each other. When obesity is caused by high amounts of blood glucose (from overeating), diabetes can result. The condition of diabetes reduces the body's ability to burn fuel, leading to obesity.

Your body's set point can be reestablished by increasing insulin sensitivity. You can do this by increasing the amount of exercise you get and eating a better diet. Whole grains and legumes, along with fresh fruit and vegetables, provide a source of carbohydrates which enter the bloodstream more gradually than refined foods. Moreover, these foods are a good source of soluble fiber, which helps slow down the release of glucose into the bloodstream. The demands of exercise will begin to reduce blood sugar levels and insulin production, eventually increasing your cells' sensitivity to insulin.

Chromium is another element that plays a key role in increasing insulin sensitivity. It ensures that insulin can transport glucose into the cells. Without it, blood sugar levels rise and thermogenesis is impaired. There has been no RDA (Recommended Dietary Allowance) established for chromium, but nutritionists feel 200 micrograms (mcg) a day are necessary for good health. Eating refined carbohydrates can lead to a deficiency of this nutrient, and there is evidence that many Americans don't get enough chromium in the foods they eat. Although there are no definitive studies showing which form of chromium is best to take, there is some indication that chromium picolinate provides the best results.

There are some people who have trouble losing weight because their sympathetic nervous system is not working correctly. This system is responsible for stimulating heart beat, dilating the pupils, and contracting the blood vessels. If it works well, the metabolism burns fuel efficiently. If this system is impaired, it becomes more difficult to keep from gaining weight.

Another factor that regulates weight loss is the activity of the pituitary gland. This gland releases growth hormone, a large molecule which regulates reproduction and other metabolic activities, as well as growth. Growth hormone is produced as we sleep and is responsible for the energy our muscles burn while we're at rest. It accounts for much of the weight we lose at night, even though we're inactive.

There are also substances in the body that are responsible for our cravings for sweets and starches. When we eat carbohydrates, the amino acid tryptophan is released into the brain. As long as the brain is getting regular amounts of tryptophan, it determines that we're getting enough to eat. If levels of tryptophan become low, the brain will send out warning signals that starvation may be imminent. In this case, we'll crave carbohydrates which provide instant energy and a quick release of more tryptophan. An imbalance of tryptophan, especially one resulting from constant dieting, can create strong urges to eat. Maintaining a constant, satisfying level of carbohydrates will keep tryptophan levels from triggering the carbohydrate cravings that can sabotage weight loss plans.

Having good sources of fiber in your diet will help you regulate your weight as well. Besides improving insulin sensitivity, fiber can help you feel more full and reduce the number of calories your body will absorb. Pectin is a good example of a water-soluble fiber that has a positive effect on weight loss. Anyone who has made jelly or jam at home is familiar with how pectin congeals when mixed with water. This same reaction takes place when pectin and water mix in the stomach, making you feel full. High-pectin foods, such as apples, help curb your appetite and increase your chances for effective weight loss. An interesting study on the effects of fiber on weight loss showed an average loss of 12.8 pounds over 4 weeks using 5.56 g of citrus pectin a day, along with a restricted-calorie diet.*

Meals with a high fat content leave you feeling full longer, because fats are often the last nutrients to be assimilated in the process of digestion. Even though you'll certainly want to watch the amount of fat in your diet, it's important to have a source of health-promoting fats. You might consider eating more of your fats in whatever meal precedes the time of day you're most likely to feel the urge to snack. If you can't get through the afternoon without a candy bar, try adding some walnuts to your lunch. If the refrigerator is your last stop before going to bed, have a large fresh salad with flax oil or olive oil for dinner.

Although being overweight is primarily a condition of too much fat in the body, water retention can contribute to the bloating that makes your clothes tighter and leaves you feeling groggy and tired. Diets high in salt are a prime contributor to water retention, but a lack of potassium can also make a difference. Potassium acts as the polar opposite of sodium; where sodium helps hold water in our body, potassium helps cells

---

*S.M. El-Shebini et al., "The Role of Pectin as a Slimming Agent," *J Clini Biochem Nutr* 4 (1988): 255-62

eliminate it. If you add more high-potassium foods to your diet, you'll be providing a better balance to the sodium in your foods. (This is not a license to go wild with the salt shaker. Don't make it a habit to reach for the salt before picking up your fork at meals.)

How does apple cider vinegar work to help you lose weight?

Dr. Jarvis was one of the first people to document the folk remedy of using apple cider vinegar for weight loss. It was generally accepted by Dr. Jarvis' Vermont patients that by taking apple cider vinegar on a regular basis, one would experience gradual, certain weight loss. The dose they used was two teaspoons in a glass of water before meals.

Although many fad diets that create rapid weight loss have come and gone over the years, it is encouraging to note that the apple cider vinegar diet leads to gradual weight loss. It would be nice if we could shed pounds quickly and never see them again, but experience has shown that weight that leaves easily comes back easily. If you lose weight quickly, your body will oblige you by kicking in mechanisms to make it more likely this weight will slip back on in no time. But if you can be patient and do not expect instant results, your fat cells will adjust to their new size more willingly and not insist on contributing to your waistline.

When you give it some thought, it makes good sense that drinking apple cider vinegar before meals would help with weight loss. We saw earlier that apples are a good source of pectin, and including pectin in your diet can make you feel fuller and more satisfied. Since apple cider vinegar contains the same amount of pectin as apples (one apple has about 1.5 grams pectin), it can suppress your appetite in a similar way.

There is also good science behind why apple cider vinegar would encourage weight loss even more effectively than eating raw apples. In general, acids help with the digestion of protein, the building blocks for some of our hormones, especially growth hormone. We've seen how this hormone is instrumental in breaking down fat cells. By increasing the acid present in your stomach before a meal, you'll ensure the chances for thorough digestion and increase the availability of protein for hormone synthesis.

Protein is needed for the production of insulin, which we know is necessary for converting glucose to energy and maintaining an active, fat-burning metabolism. Here again, apple cider vinegar can raise your metabolic rate by increasing the body's ability to utilize proteins for insulin formation.

The amino acid tryptophan plays a critical role in ensuring good levels of the neurotransmitter serotonin in the body. Serotonin is a natural mood elevator and tranquilizer. Low levels of serotonin have been linked to mental illness, especially depression, and very low levels of serotonin can sometimes lead to suicidal tendencies. As with the production of insulin, apple cider vinegar releases proteins during digestion that the body uses to build tryptophan. In this way, it begins a chain reaction that leads to a feeling of serenity and satisfaction. Because overweight can be a result of stress-induced eating, maintaining a feeling of well being can be an important factor in staying slim and healthy.

Greater protein utilization helps the formation of growth hormone, the substance that keeps the body's metabolism going while we're at rest. This is why it is important to drink apple cider vinegar before or with your evening meal. If you make sure this meal is high in protein, it will increase the amount of protein available for the apple cider vinegar to convert into amino acids. This increased protein breakdown makes it more likely that growth hormone will be produced and your metabolism will be stimulated while you sleep. (If you find a high-protein evening meal overstimulates you, consider eating it a little earlier in the evening than usual.)

Because apple cider vinegar stimulates digestion, it also reduces the amount of time that fats remain in the digestive tract. It's important that your body gets a chance to remove key nutrients from your food, and conditions that contribute to diarrhea can be life-threatening. But at the same time, it can be unhealthful to have food remain in the intestines for too long. If fats are present longer than necessary during digestion, more fats will be absorbed.

Apple cider vinegar can improve the body's utilization of iron, a nutrient that acts like firestarter for fuel. Iron is a key component in substances that carry oxygen to the cells and hold it there. Acids (like the acetic acid found in apple cider vinegar) help release iron in the food you eat and make it more available to be a building block for oxygen-carrying hemoglobin and oxygen-attracting myoglobin. Oxygen is as essential for burning energy in the body as it is for a fire to burn in a fireplace. It's the ability of apple cider vinegar to increase iron utilization and energy consumption in the body that makes it such a supportive food for weight loss. The formula for this process looks something like this:

> iron absorption ➼ oxygen utilization ➼
> energy consumption ➼ weight loss

Apple cider vinegar works at the very beginning of the digestive process to stimulate your appetite and increase your interest in food. Normally, you wouldn't think of this as being the direction you want to go in if you're trying to lose weight. But apple cider vinegar works positively to support your efforts by increasing your interest in whole foods. Vinegar is well known as a stimulator for the taste buds. It's the secret ingredient in ketchup, salad dressings, and other condiments that keeps you coming back for more. If your taste buds are working well, it's easier to appreciate the wonderful, complex flavors of whole foods such as fruits, vegetables, whole grains, and beans—all foods which will help regulate your blood sugar level and improve metabolism. You won't fall prey as easily to the tandem diet busters: salt and fat.

Apples are a great source of potassium, and likewise, apple cider vinegar, taken on a regular basis, will contribute the potassium you need to help balance the sodium in your diet. In fact, try replacing salt in your diet with apple cider vinegar. Use it to top foods you might be tempted to salt, such as vegetables or protein foods. (A little vinegar over a plate of beans is a regional favorite in many parts of America.) Salt is often present in the foods you eat as a flavor enhancer for fat. So besides increasing the amount of water weight you carry, salt can tempt you to eat more of those fatty foods—French fries, pastries, high-fat meats or meat substitutes, etc.—than you might consume otherwise.

Here is my recommendation for taking apple cider vinegar to lose weight, based on the work of Dr. Jarvis and others.

1 to 2 teaspoons apple cider vinegar + 1 glass of water *Drink before meals 3 times a day.*

If you find it difficult to drink apple cider vinegar before each meal, one glass can be taken before breakfast, one before going to bed at night, and the remaining glass drunk at sometime during the day, whenever it's convenient.

General tips for weight loss

You might find it easier to drink apple cider vinegar on a regular basis by adding it to fruit and vegetable juices. Fruit drinks will acquire a refreshing tartness, and tomato juice or mixed vegetable juice will really zing.

Besides using apple cider vinegar to increase the potassium in your diet, try incorporating other high-potassium foods to maintain the right balance of fluids in your body and prevent water retention. Great sources of potassium are mushrooms, tomatoes, potatoes, green beans, and strawberries. Contrary to popular belief, bananas are not as good a source of potassium as these other foods are.

There are many foods that are important for increasing metabolism, and perhaps none are as power packed as sea vegetables (sea weeds, such as kelp, alaria, dulse, nori, and kombu). Sea vegetables are also high in iodine, an essential element in the hormone thyroxin. Thyroxin is produced by the thyroid gland and is important for increasing the rate of metabolism in cells. Traditionally, iodized salt has been the way many Americans supplement iodine in their diets, but not all salt is iodized, including sea salt. An excellent book with information about sea vegetables and recipes for how to use them is *Sea Vegetable Celebration* by Shep Erhart and Leslie Cerier (Book Publishing Company: Summertown, Tenn.). It shows typical amounts of iodine in various sea vegetables and addresses the issue of how much iodine is too much. (Too much of a good thing can be a problem no matter what it is.)

Use whole grains as your primary snack foods, as well as your main source of carbohydrates in general. Your weight loss plan will be more successful if you can keep your blood sugar levels fairly constant, decreasing your body's cravings for quick energy boosts. Try whole grain cereals mixed with fruit juice or yogurt. (My husband was instrumental in showing me how delicious whole grain cereal is with apple juice instead of milk.) Whole grain cookies or crackers contain lots of fat and aren't going to help your cause—keep it simple. Experiment with cracked bulgur wheat or kasha (roasted buckwheat).

Other good snack ideas (especially to combat late afternoon cravings) are protein/vinegar combinations such as marinated mushrooms, tofu salad or egg salad, vegetarian sausage and mustard, vegetarian burger with catsup, and vegetarian scallops with low-fat mayonnaise and pickle relish.

The environment you create around your meals can enhance the efforts you're making to eat right. Avoid eating on the run. Slow down and give meal time your attention. It will help make you feel less like you're depriving yourself when you're cutting back on some of your favorite fattening foods. Set a nice table— invest in pretty place mats and cloth napkins, and use attractive utensils and glassware. A bowl of fruit, candles, and/or flowers will make your dinner table beautiful and inviting. Play soothing music while you eat, and if you eat alone, use this time to read a relaxing book or magazine. (My favorite is the daily crossword puzzle.) This pleasant distraction will help you eat less rapidly, allowing your body to reach a feeling of fullness on less food.

Take time after your largest meal of the day to relax, meditate, and give your body the maximum opportunity to digest your meal properly. Take a stroll, sit outdoors, lean back with a lavender-scented bag over your eyes, etc. Even a daily dose of sunshine can help stimulate your metabolism. Reclaiming your body is a healing process. Don't miss any opportunity to allow your body to operate at its best.

A word for exercise

I have to say a word here about the benefits of regular exercise as a part of any weight loss program. If all you're doing is cutting back on calories, you're doing the equivalent of just wasting away. It won't work, and the older you get, the less effective calorie restriction will be as an effective method for weight loss. Watching what you eat is important, but building up a healthy body is equally, if not more important. It's the key to building muscle that keeps on burning fat even when you're at rest. The adrenaline you generate after vigorous activity leaves you feeling energized and more interested in staying active. It also acts as a mood elevator, increasing your desire to do more. Staying active is like riding an up elevator. The more you get involved, the more you feel like staying involved.

The good news is that even a life-long couch potato can turn around a sedentary lifestyle quickly and easily. Almost everyone can walk—no athletic ability necessary—and walking has been shown to be the surest way for someone who is not physically active to get started on a fitness program. You'll feel the difference on your very first walk. Don't think you have time? Find all the opportunities you can to walk more during your usual activities. Don't burn gallons of gas trying to find the closest parking space to the door of the store. Park in the first space you come to, and walk across the parking lot. Forget escalators when you can, and take the stairs. Walk to work or the store when you can. Take the long way around to the office cafeteria or restroom. The aim here is not to save time or energy—you need to do a little more.

If you can get up a little earlier to take a long walk in the morning before work or add a walk to your evening routine, so much the better. The most successful walking program for weight loss is covering about four miles in one hour, at least five days a week (about 20 miles altogether). At that speed you can still carry on a conversation, but you'll have to swing your arms to keep up the pace.

Forget expensive gym equipment you'll never use or fancy exercise outfits—invest in really good walking shoes. Find an athletic shoe store staffed by salespeople who are knowledgeable about shoe construction and what you need in a good walking shoe. Don't wear your shoes thin. I read once that some experts feel putting 200 miles on good walking shoes is distance enough. (If you walked those 20 miles a week, they would have you buying new shoes every couple of months!) My recommendation is to watch the heels of your shoes and don't hesitate to replace them if the tread is noticeably worn down.

Create a favorable environment for walking the way you would create a pleasurable environment for eating. Find beautiful, safe places for walking—use indoor ovals as a last resort. If you can stay out of the food court, find a walker-friendly mall to use in inclement weather. If you have the room in your home, get a treadmill or ski tracker for those cold or rainy days. (Try out different models in spas or exercise rooms until you find something you really enjoy using for long periods.) If you find motivation difficult, team up with a friend. Sometimes neither I nor my walking partner will feel like getting up in the morning, but neither of us wants to disappoint the other by being a no-show.

I'd also encourage you to get instruction on using free weights (hand-held dumbbells) to build up your muscles. Lifting weights is a great complement to the workout your legs get from walking, as you can focus on your arms, pectorals, and deltoids, and use weights to increase the effectiveness of abdominal exercises. Free weights come in a great range of sizes, even down to one pound each, so you can easily find something to suit your ability. Keep them in your living room and pick them up during your favorite television show. They're much less expensive than exercise equipment and not difficult to use. There are many videos and books on using them properly.

If you think weight lifting is just for young people, I challenge you to look through a copy of the book *Growing Old Is Not for Sissies: Portraits of Senior Athletes* by Etta Clark (Pomegranate: Rohnert Park, Cal.). The many pictures of active people well into their seventies and eighties is amazing and inspiring—especially octogenarian weight lifters! Even adults in their nineties who never lifted weights before have been able to begin with light weights and add significant amounts of muscle mass.

All you have to do is start. You'll never regret it.

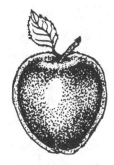

Staying Healthy with Apple Cider Vinegar

To a certain degree, good health results from a successful balance among a variety of substances in your body. Cells are constantly exchanging fluids, and the amount that is exchanged and the direction they flow are a result of how salty these fluids are. Various organs depend on the specific acidity and alkalinity of different substances in order to function properly. Apple cider vinegar is effective for health because of its role in balancing these acids and alkalines, and fluids and salts.

Understanding the acid/alkaline balance

One of the basic properties of any substance is whether it is acid or base (alkaline). In many organic processes in both plants and animals, acids and bases are formed and work to balance each other.

There are many physicians and nutrition researchers who promote theories related to the acid/alkaline balance in our bodies. Elson Hass, M.D., author of *Staying Healthy with the Seasons* and *Staying Healthy with Nutrition* (both from Celestial Arts, Berkeley), along with James Balch, M.D. and his wife Phyllis Balch, C.N.C, authors of *Prescription for Nutritional Healing* (Avery Publishing, New York) are some of the best known supporters of this concept. Although they disagree about whether it's normal for the body to be slightly acidic or alkaline (the blood is a little alkaline, the saliva a little acid), they all agree that a balance is necessary for good health. Dr. Jarvis was particularly interested in how taking regular doses of apple cider vinegar could help acid/alkaline balance.

The premise of the acid/alkaline theory states that foods create either an acid or alkaline ash when metabolized by the body. The pH (measurement of the degree of acidity or alkalinity) of this ash doesn't necessarily correspond to whether the food itself is highly acidic or not. (For example, lemons and other citrus fruit are acidic but create an alkaline ash.) It is thought that eating a diet high in meat, fats, wheat, and refined carbohydrates increases the body's acidity. This condition can lead to illness and many chronic conditions, such as insomnia, migraines, congestion, infections, and frequent colds. Alkaline-producing foods include most vegetables and fruits. Since most people eating a Western diet tend to include fewer fruits and vegetables than meat, fats, and refined foods, they have a greater problem with overacidity than overalkalinity.

Acids are essential for digestion. Hydrochloric acid mixes with enzymes in the stomach to break down protein in the foods we eat. As we age, we don't always produce the amount of hydrochloric acid we need to digest proteins properly. In fact, getting indigestion may be as much a factor of too little acid as it is too much. Taking a little apple cider vinegar before a meal helps increase stomach acidity and can improve digestion. Moreover, the malic acid and tartaric acid in apple cider vinegar deter the growth of disease-promoting bacteria in the digestive tract, protecting against food-borne pathogens. If you are digesting your foods properly, you get all the benefits of their nutrients—and feel better and stay healthier in the long run.

Minerals such as potassium, sodium, calcium, and magnesium bind to acids and neutralize them. Since fruits and vegetables are such a good source of these minerals, they play an important role in keeping the acid/alkaline balance of the body at a health-promoting level. Apple cider vinegar can help with the body's acid/alkaline balance by providing a good source of these alkalizing minerals, especially potassium.

A healthy acid/alkaline balance is also important outside the digestive system. Vinegar has long been known as an effective remedy in douches for vaginitis and yeast infections. And because the pH of apple cider vinegar approximates the slightly acidic pH of the human skin, it can help restore a pH that is out of balance due to skin problems.

Strong acids have preservative power that also relates to acid/alkaline balance. Many bacteria and molds cannot survive in a highly acidic environment. Vinegar, as well as other natural acids, have been used throughout history to preserve foods, making it a natural choice for canning and pickling. Apple cider vinegar, in particular, adds a delicious, fruity flavor to pickles, relish, and other preserves.

Understanding the fluid/salt balance

Another important equation in the interplay of body chemistry is between salty fluids and water. It's a basic fact of biochemistry that if you have a salty solution on one side of a membrane and water on the other, the water will be drawn in the direction of the salt solution. A common example of this effect is the drying and curing of meats with salt.

Sodium and potassium salts perform a balancing act on either side of our cell walls. Without potassium, the sodium solutions outside our cells would draw water out of the cells, and we'd eventually dry up. A complex chemical process exchanges potassium from our extracellular (outside the cell) fluids with sodium that might be in our cells. Our bodies are able to balance the water-absorbing sodium that circulates by holding onto some counteracting potassium as long as we have a good supply of potassium in our diets. Potassium and sodium also move back and forth through nerve cells to regulate the heartbeat and help muscles contract.

Sodium in the form of sodium chloride (table salt) was once a scarce commodity in our diet. We now "enjoy" a state of dietary affluence where salt is plentiful, but our body chemistry has not evolved to keep up with this affluence. The marked increase in our salt consumption from prehistoric times has resulted in a two-fold increase in our average sodium intake. Unfortunately, at the same time, our consumption of potassium has dropped. Higher levels of sodium cause more water to be drawn out of the cells, increasing the fluid level in the bloodstream and raising blood pressure.

The presence of potassium in our cells makes it more difficult for bacteria to draw moisture from the cells in order to grow and multiply. Because it works to keeps water in our cells, potassium helps keeps tissues soft. Potassium also draws excess water out of the body by moving it to the kidneys.

Potassium is very important for proper metabolism, as it affects the utilization of protein and carbohydrates. Unfortunately we have a more difficult time absorbing and retaining potassium as we get older. A potassium deficiency causes lack of cell growth, or, in some cases, abnormal growth. This can result in fatigue, muscle weakness, dry skin or acne, insomnia, elevated blood sugar, and heart rhythm disturbances. Severe deficiencies can lead to fragile bones, kidney problems, and changes in the central nervous system.

On pages 29 and 33 we talked how potassium helps prevent water weight gain. Here we see that its protective qualities are numerous and diverse, making it an important nutrient to include in our diet. Apple cider vinegar is a good source of potassium, providing 15 mg per tablespoon, as well as other important minerals (see page 19).

Apple cider vinegar - your personal medicine box

Among the experts on apple cider vinegar, there is general agreement on the usefulness of a tonic made by **adding 1 to 2 teaspoons of apple cider vinegar to a glass of water and drinking this before or during each meal**. You can try this simple formula to start experiencing the benefits of apple cider vinegar in your diet. Experiment with the amount of vinegar you add until you find a level that works for you. Some people also recommend adding a teaspoon of honey to this mixture; depending on your dietary needs and preferences, this is entirely up to you. And by all means, sip this tonic slowly and leisurely; it will be better tolerated and more effective if you don't gulp it down.

If you find that drinking this tonic before or during meals is upsetting to your stomach, try it a little while after a meal. If your meal schedule does not make it practical to take a tonic when you eat, try having a glass as you're getting dressed in the morning, another just before going to bed, and the third glass at some other time during the day.

On the following pages are remedies for specific conditions.

APPLE CIDER VINEGAR FOR COMMON AILMENTS

Besides providing a general health benefit, there are many tried and true folk remedies using apple cider vinegar for specific conditions that you might find useful. Here is a compilation.

acne – Grate 1 pound of horseradish and combine with 2 cups of apple cider vinegar. Let sit for 2 weeks, then strain. Apply the liquid to acne spots daily with a cotton ball.

aging, premature – This can be a sign that your metabolism is not operating efficiently. Take 2 teaspoons of apple cider vinegar with 2 teaspoons of honey in a glass of water daily.

allergies – Regular use of apple cider vinegar can help with allergies by generally strengthening the immune system and improving metabolism.

arthritis – Although there is no definitive research on whether apple cider vinegar will cure arthritis, there are many people who will attest to its effectiveness. There are a variety of formulas for using apple cider vinegar for arthritis, ranging from 2 to as many as 10 teaspoons taken with water at meals until the pain subsides. In addition to using apple cider vinegar, it is also advised to maintain a healthy weight, don't smoke, and be sure to include a variety of vegetables in the diet. Arthritis can be aggravated by food allergies, so you may want to consider removing foods that contain wheat, dairy, corn, and citrus from your diet, one group at a time, and see if eliminating any one of them makes a difference.

asthma – If you have mild asthma, try drinking a general tonic along with applying a vinegar-soaked compress to the insides of your wrists. For asthma that occasionally keeps you up at night, sip a glass of water containing 1 tablespoon of apple cider vinegar over the course of half an hour. If wheezing persists half an hour after that, try another dose (although usually breathing difficulties will have subsided by then).

athlete's foot – Try soaking the feet twice a day in a mixture of half apple cider vinegar-half water, or apply pure apple cider vinegar directly to affected areas of the foot several times during the day and before bedtime.

> ### The Apple Cider Vinegar Tonic
>
> 1 to 2 teaspoons apple cider vinegar
>
> +
>
> 1 glass of water
>
> Drink before or during meals 3 times a day.

bladder and kidney problems, bladder infections – Patricia Bragg recommends this healing and cleansing drink: 2 tablespoons fresh or dried corn silk to 1 quart distilled water or marshmallow herbal tea. (The marshmallow here is an herb, not the sugary gelatin confection.) Take 1 cup, 2 to 3 times daily, with ½ teaspoon apple cider vinegar and a teaspoon of buckwheat honey added.

bleeding – Vinegar has been used by physicians up until the last century to treat wounds and stop bleeding. Dr. Jarvis believed the adrenaline-like effect of apple cider vinegar helped it to coagulate blood.

A cotton ball soaked with apple cider vinegar makes a good remedy for nosebleeds. Placing this in the bleeding nostril will help staunch the nosebleed more quickly than using a plain cotton ball. Have the person lay their head back in order to use the force of gravity in reversing the blood flow.

Apple cider vinegar taken as a general tonic is good for someone right before and after surgery (with the exception of intestinal surgery).

blood pressure – Take the general tonic to gain the benefits of potassium in apple cider vinegar. Potassium helps balance sodium in the body and lowers blood pressure.

bone health – Apple cider vinegar contains minerals such as magnesium, manganese, and silicon, all of which contribute to good health. It also contains the trace mineral boron which supports the metabolism of calcium and magnesium for making strong bones. In addition, boron helps elevate levels of estrogen and testosterone, which helps keep bones strong. Taking the general apple cider vinegar tonic will provide a good source of these minerals.

breathing problems – *(see asthma)*

bruises – Dissolve 1 teaspoon salt in ½ cup apple cider vinegar. Heat this mixture slightly and apply to the bruise as a compress.

burns – Use full-strength apple cider vinegar to reduce the pain of burns, even sunburns.

cancer – Apple cider vinegar contains a number of substances that protect against cancer. Beta-carotene is a powerful antioxidant that helps fight the effect of free radicals in the body. Pectin, found in cider and the skins of apples, binds to free radicals and keeps food from stagnating in the colon, thus decreasing the release of potential toxins. Take the apple cider vinegar tonic regularly to get a good supply of pectin in your diet.

An interesting research finding shows that vinegar can be very effective (and perhaps even more effective than a regular Pap smear) at detecting cervical cancer. A study was published several years ago in *The Lancet* by researchers at Johns Hopkins University in Baltimore and the University of Zimbabwe. In the study, nurse midwives screened almost 11,000 women in Zimbabwe for cervical cancer using both acetic acid (the primary ingredient in vinegar) and the traditional pap smear. Researchers indicated that "the vinegar test was more likely to pick up precancerous or cancerous cells than the pap smear."

> ### The Apple Cider Vinegar Tonic
>
> I to 2 teaspoons apple cider vinegar
>
> +
>
> I glass of water
>
> Drink before or during meals 3 times a day.

canker sores – Relieve canker sores by rinsing the mouth with 1 teaspoon of apple cider vinegar in a glass of water several times a day until healed.

candida – *(see yeast)*

cataracts – Cataracts can result from damage to the lens of the eye and are a common problem of aging. Studies have shown that people with a diet high in beta-carotene and vitamins C and E (all of which are present in apple cider vinegar) are less likely to get cataracts. Take the general tonic for optimum protection. It's important to note that diets high in salt and fat increase the risk for cataracts.

chicken pox – Relieve the discomfort of chicken pox by applying full-strength apple cider vinegar to affected areas, and add 1 cup to a warm bath.

cholesterol – Pectin is a soluble fiber which absorbs fats and cholesterol and removes them from the body. Taking apple cider vinegar either in the morning or throughout the day as a tonic is an effective way to be sure you have a source of pectin in your diet. Also, the amino acids in apple cider vinegar can neutralize harmful oxidized LDL cholesterol.

cold sores – You can relieve the discomfort of cold sores and herpes sores and decrease the amount of time needed to heal them by applying full-strength apple cider vinegar directly on the sores until they subside.

colds – Your body is more alkaline during a cold. A teaspoon of apple cider vinegar in half a cup of water taken several times a day at the onset of a cold can help your acid/alkaline balance and boost your body's own healing powers. For a cold accompanied by nasal congestion, try breathing in a steam vapor made by heating a mixture of half apple cider vinegar and half water. Not only will the vinegar vapors help open nasal passages, the moisture from the steam will help retard the activity of the viruses that cause colds. And then there's the time-honored folk remedy of soaking brown paper (you can cut up a paper bag) in vinegar, then sprinkling the paper with a little black pepper. Place the paper on the chest with the peppered side toward the skin, cover with a towel, and leave on for 20 minutes. Be sure to keep the cold sufferer warm.

constipation – Constipation can be caused by poor diet, as well as the normal reduction of digestive acids we experience as we age. Constipation can be a serious problem, as it increases the length of time that toxins remain in the colon and slows down the flow of nutrients the body absorbs. Eating a diet rich in fiber is the most natural and effective way to combat constipation, and apple cider vinegar is a good source of water-soluble pectin. Either try the daily tonic or the following flax and vinegar recipe from Patricia Bragg: Boil 2 cups distilled water and ¼ cup flaxseed for 10 minutes. (It will become gelatinous as it cools.) Take 2 tablespoons of this mixture and combine it with 1 teaspoon apple cider vinegar. Drink it when you get up in the morning and again one hour after dinner.

corns – Soak feet in a warm water bath with ¼ to ½ cup apple cider vinegar added. Rub the corns with a pumice stone, apply full-strength apple cider vinegar directly to the corn, cover with a bandage, and leave on overnight. Apply vinegar and a bandage again in the morning. Repeat until the corn has dissolved.

> ## The Apple Cider Vinegar Tonic
>
> 1 to 2 teaspoons apple cider vinegar
>
> +
>
> 1 glass of water
>
> Drink before or during meals 3 times a day.

coughs – One of the oldest and most familiar home remedies for a cough is a combination of honey and lemon juice. You can substitute apple cider vinegar for the lemon juice, combining twice as much honey as vinegar. Take anywhere from 1 teaspoon to 1 tablespoon of this mixture at a time, 5 to 6 times a day, especially right before bed when nighttime coughing can disrupt your sleep. This remedy is especially good for children, who can sometimes get an upset stomach from over-the-counter cough syrups.

Another folk remedy for coughing spells at night is sprinkling apple cider vinegar on your pillow case or a cloth placed on the pillow.

cramps – *(see also leg cramps)* Muscle cramps can be caused by a deficiency of vitamin E in the diet or an imbalance of calcium and magnesium in the body. Taking apple cider vinegar regularly as a tonic will supply helpful minerals and vitamin E.

cuts and abrasions – Apple cider vinegar has been used to heal wounds for centuries. Applying it full strength will not only reduce the chance of infection but will also increase the speed of healing.

dandruff – Using apple cider vinegar full strength on your scalp will help destroy the bacteria and/or fungus that causes dandruff. Apply to the scalp, rub in, and leave on for a half hour to an hour before washing your hair.

depression – Depression can range from an occasional mood problem to a serious metabolic disorder. Although the severity and causes vary widely with each individual, some Eastern medicine practices subscribe to the belief that depression is caused by a stagnant liver. A daily dose of apple cider vinegar works as a liver-cleansing tonic, helped by the amino acids it contains. Since mood can be influenced by the level of serotonin in the brain, apple cider vinegar can help there as well. *(see page 31)*

diabetes – Diabetes results when the body is no longer able to properly process blood glucose. A daily tonic of apple cider vinegar can supply pectin, a water-soluble fiber good for helping to regulate glucose levels. Since many diabetes sufferers have impaired digestive functions, apple cider vinegar can also help restore good digestion and nutrient absorption. *(see page 51)*

diaper rash – Apple cider vinegar is an effective cure for many forms of rashes caused by fungus and bacteria. Use half-strength as a remedy for diaper rash.

diarrhea – Diarrhea can be caused by harmful bacteria in the colon. Not only will apple cider vinegar help the body get rid of harmful bacteria, but the pectin in it will also help to absorb water in the intestines and provide more bulk for the stool. Take the daily tonic, but divide it into six doses and sip it slowly. Diarrhea that persists for a couple of days or is severe can be a serious health problem, and you should contact your health care provider immediately.

digestion, burping – One of the most important contributions apple cider vinegar makes to our health and well being is to enhance digestion. This contribution begins in the mouth with the stimulation of saliva. Acid receptors on the tongue begin a strong flow of saliva when they come in contact with vinegar, starting a digestive process that begins the breakdown of carbohydrates. Apple cider vinegar also enhances the action of hydrochloric acid and digestive enzymes in the stomach. Anyone who is making significant changes in their diet might be helped by sipping $\frac{1}{3}$ cup water with 1 teaspoon apple cider vinegar 3 times a day. Vinegar's antibacterial properties can help digestive acids reduce the opportunity for bacterial infection in the stomach, so world travelers might be well served by taking along a small bottle of apple cider vinegar in their suitcases. Finally, vinegar can also ameliorate the effects of a large, rich dinner eaten late in the evening by promoting the breakdown of foods that might otherwise linger for hours in the digestive tract.

> **The Apple Cider Vinegar Tonic**
>
> 1 to 2 teaspoons apple cider vinegar
> +
> 1 glass of water
>
> Drink before or during meals 3 times a day.

dizziness – Dizziness can result from an alkaline condition in the body, as well as a number of conditions that affect the central nervous system by sending conflicting information from the eyes, ears, etc. Many people find relief from dizziness by taking the apple cider vinegar tonic on a regular basis.

ear aches – Infections in any part of the ear require the attention of a physician. But while you're waiting for medical care or the effects of antibiotics to take hold, try holding the affected ear over a steam bath of 1 part apple cider vinegar to 2 parts water. (Be sure the ear is not so close to the source of the steam that it gets burned.) This seems like a good remedy for young children who get frequent ear infections, as it provides relief from pain, as well as healing benefits.

eczema – Use apple cider vinegar diluted with equal amounts of water to relieve the itching and dryness of eczema.

exhaustion – Exhaustion in and of itself is not a serious medical condition, but it can have a temporary, debilitating effect on your performance and well being. Try a refreshing apple cider vinegar sponge bath, using it full strength and allowing it to remain on the skin until it dries in the air.

fatigue – The amino acids in apple cider vinegar can neutralize the build-up of lactic acid in the bloodstream that occurs after exercise and stress. It's also thought that the enzymes and amino acids one gets through regular use of a vinegar tonic can help beat fatigue.

fever – Vinegar compresses to the lower legs have been recommended by physicians for years to reduce fever. While keeping the person with the fever warm, wrap their calves with tea towels soaked in 1 part apple cider vinegar and 3 parts water. Resoak and apply the compresses when they become dry. A similar folk remedy involves soaking cotton socks in this solution and placing them back on the feet, wrapping the feet in towels to keep them warm.

flatulence – Flatulence is a result of the incomplete digestion of carbohydrates, especially those that occur in foods like beans and cabbage. If flatulence is a problem, try sipping a glass of apple cider vinegar tonic before meals.

food poisoning – The antibacterial action of apple cider vinegar makes it a good remedy for fighting off the harmful bacteria that cause food poisoning. Take very small sips from 2 glasses of apple cider vinegar tonic over an 8-hour period. Drink only clear fluids like tea, club soda, or water—no fruit juices or sugary sodas. You can also use a vinegar tonic as a preventative if you're eating in foreign countries or at picnics, anywhere the food might not be properly prepared or refrigerated.

> ### The Apple Cider Vinegar Tonic
>
> I to 2 teaspoons apple cider vinegar
> +
> I glass of water
>
> Drink before or during meals 3 times a day.

foot care – If you've had a hard day on your feet and they're swollen and sore, try a refreshing foot bath. Add several cups of apple cider vinegar to a basin of warm water, and soak for 15 to 20 minutes. Remove your feet and air dry to increase the cooling effects. (*see also athlete's foot*)

fungus infections – (*see also diaper rash*) Use a solution of half apple cider vinegar and half water several times a day on fungus infections until cleared.

gallbladder, gallstones – Apple cider vinegar can be used as part of a popular alternative treatment known as a gallbladder flush. There are many variations on this, but basically whole apples, apple juice, applesauce, and/or apple cider vinegar tonic are the only foods or beverages consumed for 2 to 3 days. At the end of this period, straight olive oil is drunk at bedtime. Some practitioners combine olive oil with apple juice or cider vinegar, especially for routine removal of small gallstones that are not causing discomfort. Sometimes an enema is prescribed for the morning following the ingestion of the olive oil. The common result is the flushing of very small gallstones with the enema or next bowel movement. While painful gallstones should be treated by a physician, an annual gallbladder flush can help avoid the formation of larger stones. The efficacy of this treatment can be substantiated by the relative lack of gallbladder problems in people who are regular apple cider vinegar users.

gums, bleeding – Apple cider vinegar tonic can be used as a mouth rinse for bleeding gums. The action of vinegar dissolves plaque that can aggravate gums and helps fight oral infections much in the same way it does with cuts and scrapes.

headaches – There is general agreement among apple cider vinegar experts that headaches are a result of too much alkalinity in the body. The fastest way to get relief from a headache is to try a little apple cider vinegar aromatherapy by breathing in the steam from cider vinegar vapors. Use either several tablespoons of cider vinegar simmered in 2 quarts of water or equal parts of water and cider vinegar. Lean over the simmering water, being careful not to breathe so closely down into the steam that it burns your mucus membranes. You can use a towel over your head to help direct the steam towards you. Adding cider vinegar to a vaporizer can also provide relief. If you're somewhere where the steam treatment is not practical, you might get relief from breathing the vapors from a small bottle of apple cider vinegar. If you have frequent stress headaches, you might consider keeping a small bottle in your purse or desk drawer.

head lice – If you find that over-the-counter lice preparations are too toxic to your skin, try rinsing your hair with full-strength apple cider vinegar. Do not wash it out, but wrap your head with a scarf and leave it in until the next time you wash your hair. Use for 2 to 3 days in order to kill adult lice. There is no better way to completely get rid of head lice than by killing the adult lice, then examining each strand of hair in good sunlight on three consecutive days so you can strip off the lice eggs that remain with your finger nails. Lice combs won't do a thorough enough job, and the eggs are too difficult to see in artificial light.

heartburn – (see indigestion)

> ### The Apple Cider Vinegar Tonic
>
> 1 to 2 teaspoons apple cider vinegar
> +
> 1 glass of water
>
> Drink before or during meals 3 times a day.

hemorrhoids – The healing properties of full strength apple cider vinegar applied directly to hemorrhoids can reduce stinging and promote shrinking. Regular use of the apple cider vinegar tonic can help soften stools and reduce the need for straining during elimination. This will help prevent hemorrhoids in the first place.

herpes – (see cold sores)

hiccups – There are as many remedies for hiccups as there are hiccup sufferers, so it's no surprise that cider vinegar experts have offered a couple of options. Either slowly sip a glass of warm apple cider vinegar tonic (preferably from the far side of the glass), or take 1 tablespoon of cider vinegar mixed with 1 tablespoon refined sugar. (This is one instance where refined sugar can be used as a remedy.)

hives and rashes – Try mixing equal parts of apple cider vinegar and cornstarch to make a paste you can apply to hives and rashes. This combination will help calm the itching.

hoarseness – (see sore throat)

impetigo (staph/strep infections) – Impetigo is the result of either a streptococcus or staphylococcus infection of the skin and is especially contagious and troublesome in young children, who tend to touch everything. Apply full strength apple cider vinegar to the skin every 3 hours; you should see results in several days. If it is a severe case, or if there is danger of widespread contagion, you should consult your physician.

indigestion, heartburn – Indigestion and heartburn result from too little hydrochloric acid in the stomach as often as they do from too much acid in the stomach or the movement of acid into the esophagus. Regular use of apple cider vinegar tonic helps break down protein and fats in the stomach. It is especially effective if taken before a large meal, as it stimulates the flow of saliva that promotes digestion. Try using this remedy instead of antacid tablets. Regular use of antacids can provide immediate relief, but they will decrease the acid content of the stomach and possibly intensify the discomfort they were meant to alleviate.

insect bites and stings – Use full-strength apple cider vinegar on a variety of insect bites and stings, including bee stings, fire ants, mosquitoes, wasp stings, and spider bites. (Be sure to get appropriate treatment for brown recluse spider bites and immediate medical care if you are allergic to bee or wasp stings.) You can also use it to reduce the pain of jellyfish stings, so take apple cider vinegar with you if you are vacationing in beach areas where jellyfish frequent.

insomnia – If you have difficulty going to sleep at night, try a glass of apple cider vinegar tonic with a little honey added before bed time. Keep another glass ready in case you wake up during the night. The carbohydrates in both the cider vinegar and honey will activate serotonin, a brain chemical that promotes relaxation.

jellyfish stings – *(see insect bites)*

jock itch – As with other rashes, use a mixture of half apple cider vinegar and half water applied directly to relieve the itching.

kidney stones – *(see gallbladder)*

lameness – A favorite remedy for soreness in the legs comes from Dr. Jarvis: 1 tablespoon apple cider vinegar combined with the yolk of 1 egg and 1 tablespoon turpentine. Apply daily to the legs as needed.

The Apple Cider Vinegar Tonic
1 to 2 teaspoons apple cider vinegar
+
1 glass of water
Drink before or during meals 3 times a day.

laryngitis – *(see sore throat)*

leg cramps – Regular use of the apple cider vinegar tonic can help the absorption of calcium and magnesium which can protect against frequent, painful leg cramps, especially at night.

liver function – Apple cider vinegar has long been considered a detoxifying substance, so it would make sense that it would promote the activities of one of our major toxin-eliminating organs, the liver.

To promote good liver function, bump up the amount of apple cider vinegar in your daily tonic to 1 tablespoon. This will help to break down fats and proteins from rich foods that can tax the liver.

longevity – A deterioration in your appearance may be more a factor of poor metabolism than aging. Taking the apple cider vinegar tonic on a regular basis can improve digestion and increase metabolism, resulting in better skin tone, less joint pain, improved memory, and a trimmer figure.

memory – Apple cider vinegar helps the body metabolize iron and provides trace amounts of amino acids. Iron helps move oxygen to the cells, and amino acids are necessary for the synthesis of brain chemicals; both of these factors help improve memory. Many experts feel that people who use cider vinegar regularly in the diet have consistently good mental powers long into their later years.

menstrual problems – A morning glass of apple cider vinegar tonic can help reduce the flow of a heavy period. If drinking the tonic daily makes your period late, stop taking it about 3 to 4 days before you expect your period to start.

morning sickness – Just as indigestion can be a problem of too little stomach acid, rather than too much, the nausea of morning sickness can occur because the stomach has had no stimulus to make digestive acids after a night of inactivity. Sometimes the best cure for not wanting to eat anything is to eat a little of something. Sipping a little apple cider vinegar tonic can help bring about a comfortable balance of stomach acids.

Sometimes nausea can be alleviated by cooling the body. Some experts recommend a compress soaked in apple cider vinegar and applied to the stomach in order to cool the area that's most in distress.

muscle soreness, stiff joints – Apply apple cider vinegar directly to sore muscles and stiff joints to relieve pain. It can also be used to soak compresses or added to a bath to ease joint and muscle pain. Taking the daily apple cider vinegar tonic will help supply potassium to correct the mineral imbalance that might be contributing to aching joints.

nasal congestion – (see colds)

nausea – (see morning sickness)

nettles – (see poison ivy)

nervous tic – Drinking an apple cider vinegar tonic can help provide minerals that regulate the nervous system.

neuralgia, facial – This painful condition can often be remedied by sipping a mixture of equal parts apple cider vinegar and water to rectify the alkaline condition that causes neuralgia.

> ### The Apple Cider Vinegar Tonic
>
> I to 2 teaspoons apple cider vinegar
>
> +
>
> I glass of water
>
> Drink before or during meals 3 times a day.

night sweats – For night sweats that are a result of a waning cold or flu, try an apple vinegar sponge bath before going to bed. This might be a good remedy for menopausal women whose night sweats are caused by normal hormonal rebalancing during this time of their lives. Drinking a glass of cider vinegar tonic in the morning can help regulate toxins that the body is trying to eliminate through perspiration.

nosebleeds – (see bleeding)

poison ivy and poison oak (also nettles) – As with other itching, rashes, and insect bites, apple cider vinegar works quickly to relieve discomfort. Mix equal parts of cider vinegar and water, and apply directly. Patricia Bragg recommends keeping a spray bottle of this in the refrigerator, because the cool temperature of the spray provides even more relief.

pyelitis, inflammation of the kidneys – Dr. Jarvis claimed he had good results treating pyelitis using the daily apple cider vinegar tonic. As with any serious medical condition, a kidney infection should receive immediate care by your physician. The cider vinegar tonic would be a good choice to supplement your doctor's treatment if your inflammation tends to be chronic.

rashes – (see hives and rashes)

shingles – Shingles is a painful condition of the nerves of the skin. Dr. Jarvis advised applying full-strength apple cider vinegar directly to the areas of discomfort 6 to 8 times during a 24-hour period (through the night as well). This may cause a little itching and burning which will pass quickly, and it will promote better healing in the long run.

sinusitis – Try taking a glass of the apple cider vinegar tonic each hour for 6 to 8 hours to relieve sinusitis caused by too much alkalinity in the body.

sore throat (also laryngitis) – Remedies for sore throat using apple cider vinegar range from the dose in the cider vinegar tonic to using equal parts vinegar and water. In either case, do not swallow this rinse. You don't want to keep ingesting the germs that are causing the infection. Use this as a gargle or rinse hourly until symptoms subside. This is a good treatment for laryngitis or a preventative if you're going to be putting a lot of stress on your throat. It can reduce swelling and the flow of mucus.

sunburn and windburn – (see burns)

swimmer's ear – Combine the drying effect of alcohol with the disinfecting quality of apple cider vinegar for reducing the itching and pain of swimmer's ear. Use 3 to 4 drops in the ears after swimming or showering.

thrush – (see fungus)

tinnitus – Tinnitus is an annoying condition that results in constant ringing in the ears; it may have a variety of causes. A daily apple cider vinegar tonic helps improve circulation and mineral balance, both of which can have a positive effect.

tooth decay – (see also gums, bleeding) A daily rinse with a glass of apple cider vinegar tonic can help maintain good oral hygiene and fight the bacteria that lead to tooth decay and gum disease.

The Apple Cider Vinegar Tonic
1 to 2 teaspoons apple cider vinegar
+
1 glass of water
Drink before or during meals 3 times a day.

ulcers – Preliminary studies have shown that a weak concentration of vinegar can help stimulate the digestive system to combat alcohol-induced ulcers. More work in this area may show that apple cider vinegar can help prevent ulcers from forming.

urinary problems – (see also bladder) Drinking an apple cider vinegar tonic regularly before meals can help regulate urine production and protect the kidneys from infection.

varicose veins – A number of apple cider vinegar experts recommend soaking a compress in cider vinegar and wrapping it around the legs twice a day for a month. Keep the legs elevated for about half an hour before removing the compress. Also drink the cider vinegar tonic before or with meals.

warts – Combine 1 part salt with 4 parts apple cider vinegar, and apply several times a day to warts until they disappear.

yeast infections – Use a douche of 2 tablespoons apple cider vinegar and 1 quart warm water twice a day until the burning and itching of a yeast infection has stopped. You can also add a cup of cider vinegar to your bath to provide external relief.

A nutritious diet for health

You can pair up apple cider vinegar with a variety of nutritious foods to get a super health boost. Onions can help reduce asthma, and garlic is useful for fighting infection and cancer. Together they have been shown to reduce blood sugar in people with diabetes and lower blood pressure in people with hypertension. In areas of the world where olive oil is the primary source of fat, heart disease is relatively low. Cruciferous vegetables are real nutritional powerhouses; cabbage can help heal stomach ulcers, kale can protect eyes from macular degeneration, and broccoli (particularly broccoli sprouts) may be an especially effective cancer fighter. The lycopene in tomatoes may protect men against prostate cancer, and soy protein has been shown to protect against heart disease.

I hope you'll check the recipes in this book for new and delicious ways to use apple cider vinegar. You'll find many dishes that combine it with some of the foods previously mentioned, so you'll get the additional benefit of many powerful nutrients working together to bring you renewed vigor and good health.

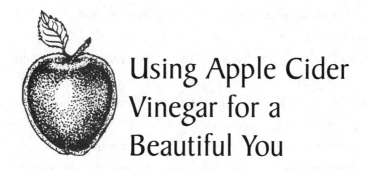

Using Apple Cider Vinegar for a Beautiful You

Besides being an effective tool for weight loss and an important remedy in your medicine cabinet, apple cider vinegar is also a great cosmetic aid. The surface of your skin is slightly acidic, but the use of soaps can make it more alkaline. In order to help your skin maintain its protective qualities, you can use apple cider vinegar in a number of ways that are not only healthful, but leave you looking more beautiful and radiant as well.

In the bath

The easiest way to do this is to use apple cider vinegar when you shower or bathe. Try adding 1 to 2 cups to your next bath instead of using soap. (This is also a good remedy for sore muscles, and the combination of moist heat and vinegar is very soothing.) Keep a plastic bottle of apple cider vinegar in your shower stall, and apply it to your skin either with your cupped hands or on a wash cloth. You'll be surprised at the clean, refreshing tingle you'll feel. Apple cider vinegar is also an effective deodorant, because it provides an acid barrier that fights bacteria and other oder-causing germs. Instead of relying on perfumed soaps and deodorants that can irritate skin, neutralize the organisms that cause body odor and leave your skin with a fresh, clean scent.

Whether or not you choose to use apple cider vinegar when you bathe, be sure to try it as part of a gentle massage to invigorate tired skin and give it a healthy glow. Add about ¼ cup to several quarts of water, and apply it to your skin with a wash cloth, gently rubbing the skin with a circular motion.

You can also make apple cider vinegar a part of a regular facial to help remove dead cells and prevent acne and other skin blemishes. Make a steam facial by covering your head with a towel and bending over a bowl of very hot water to which you've added ½ cup apple cider vinegar. Use a cleansing pad or wash cloth to wipe your face and remove dirt and oil. Be sure to finish with a splash of cold water to close pores.

You can also open up your pores by rinsing out a hand towel in hot water and covering your face with it for a few minutes. Remove the hand towel and cover your face with a tea towel soaked in 1 quart warm water to which several tablespoons of apple cider vinegar have been added. Place on top of that another application of a warmed hand towel for several minutes. Remove all the towels and finish by rubbing your face with a clean, wet wash cloth to stimulate your skin and remove dead cells and oils.

Hair care

While you're bathing, don't forget to use the classic application of apple cider vinegar as a natural rinse for loosening tangles and restoring the natural luster and shine to tired, damaged hair. Add ¼ cup of apple cider vinegar to 1 quart warm water, and use as a final rinse. This mixture will also help fight the bacteria that cause dandruff.

Feet and legs

Apple cider vinegar can be used to make you more beautiful from head to toe, so don't neglect your feet. You can use it to invigorate tired feet, reduce foot oder and athlete's foot, and treat corns and calluses. For a refreshing foot soak, add ¼ to ½ cup apple cider vinegar to a basin of lukewarm water, and soak your feet for about 10 minutes daily. This will help destroy the bacteria that cause foot odor and the fungus that leads to athlete's foot. For corns and callouses, use the greater amount of apple cider vinegar and increase the soaking time to about half an hour. You can then use a pumice stone (look for them anywhere foot care products are sold) to rub away any corns and callouses.

If you use nail polish frequently, try rubbing clean nails with a cotton ball saturated with apple cider vinegar before applying polish. The vinegar will remove any residual oils on the nails and help the polish stay on longer. It will also promote healthy nails and cuticles.

Finally, many of us will develop varicose veins in our legs as we get older. As an alternative to expensive treatments for removing these unsightly veins, try this folk remedy: Soak tea towels in apple cider vinegar, and use them to wrap your legs. Elevate your legs and leave the towels on for half an hour. Do this twice a day for at least six weeks to get results. Also use the apple cider vinegar tonic from page 43 to increase the effectiveness of this remedy.

You can have the same beautiful glow as a polished apple, without the chemicals and expense of commercial cosmetics, by dipping into nature's beauty secret: apple cider vinegar.

Remember too that your real beauty comes from inside, and a healthy, balanced system that is regularly cleansed and fortified with apple cider vinegar can really make you shine.

Cooking with Apple Cider Vinegar

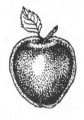

Recipes for healthy eating

Marinated Mushrooms

10 servings

The combination of mushrooms with apple cider vinegar makes this appetizer especially high in potassium.

⅓ cup apple cider vinegar
⅓ cup olive oil
4 tablespoons chopped fresh parsley
1 tablespoon salt
1 tablespoon brown sugar
1 teaspoon prepared mustard
1 small onion, sliced
1 pound fresh mushrooms (best if somewhat
   on the small side)

Combine everything except the onions and mushrooms, and bring to a boil. Add the onion slices and whole mushrooms, and refrigerate overnight.

Marinated Vegetables

10 servings

This makes a wonderful party appetizer.

Have ready:

6 to 8 cups of a mixture of your favorite vegetables, cut in bite-size pieces (You can use cauliflower, artichoke hearts, olives, bell peppers, mushrooms, carrots, zucchini, or cucumber. Cherry tomatoes and red bell peppers are nice for their color.)

Marinade

1½ cups olive oil
⅔ cup apple cider vinegar
2 teaspoons salt
1 teaspoon freshly ground black pepper
2 cloves garlic
⅓ cup sugar

Place all the veggies, except the cherry tomatoes, in a large bowl. Mix the marinade ingredients, pour over the prepared vegetables, and refrigerate. (There won't be enough marinade to cover the vegetables, but that's alright.) Stir the mixture several times a day for 3 days so that all the vegetables will be sitting in the marinade from time to time. Add any cherry tomatoes on the last day. Before serving, remove the garlic cloves and drain the vegetables. Serve with toothpicks.

Sweet-Sour Slaw

10 servings

1 medium cabbage, shredded
1 large onion, diced
1 green bell pepper, diced
1 red bell pepper, diced
1 (4-ounce) jar diced pimientos
1 cup apple cider vinegar
½ cup canola oil
½ cup sweetener of your choice
½ teaspoon turmeric
1 teaspoon celery seed
½ teaspoon salt

Combine the cabbage, onion, pepper, and pimientos in a large bowl. Mix the vinegar, canola oil, sweetener, turmeric, celery seed, and salt in a jar; cover and shake well. Pour the mixture over the vegetables, and toss lightly.

Colorful Vegetable Slaw

6 to 8 servings

I like slaws that have other vegetables besides cabbage and carrots added, both for their eye appeal as well as their nutritional value.

5 cups finely shredded green cabbage

2 cups finely shredded red cabbage

2 cups minced broccoli flowerettes

I carrot, coarsely grated

2 tablespoons minced onion

2 tablespoons sliced red bell pepper

Dressing

⅔ cup canola oil

⅓ cup apple cider vinegar

2 teaspoons Dijon mustard

I teaspoon sugar (optional)

½ teaspoon salt

Combine all the vegetables in a bowl. Mix the dressing ingredients, pour over the vegetables, and toss. This is best if left to refrigerate a few hours before serving.

Pear Salad

4 servings

This unusual salad is the perfect opener for a memorable meal.

I large bunch watercress or arugula
3 ripe pears
I avocado

Dressing

½ cup canola oil
3 tablespoons apple cider vinegar
2 teaspoons sugar or other granulated sweetener
¼ teaspoon salt
I tablespoon tomato paste

Wash and remove the stems from the watercress or arugula. Combine the dressing ingredients and set aside. Peel the pears and avocado, and slice them thinly. (Place the slices in cold salted water to prevent discoloration if it will be a little while before you're ready to serve the salad.) Rinse the pear and avocado slices well, and arrange them over the greens on salad plates. Add the dressing and serve immediately.

German Potato Salad

8 servings

This traditional favorite comes from an old Mennonite recipe.

4 pounds potatoes (about 8 cups sliced)
3 cups chopped onion
2 tablespoons sweetener of your choice
Salt and pepper, to taste
¼ cup vegetarian bacon bits
¾ cup hot water
¾ cup cider vinegar

Boil the potatoes until tender. Peel and slice them while warm. Add the onions, sweetener, salt, and pepper. Soak the bacon bits in the hot water and vinegar until just starting to soften. Pour over the potatoes and onions, and toss lightly.

Mixed Marinated Beans

10 servings

This is a great dish for pot lucks or to have around for hot summer suppers.

I pound frozen green beans, cooked and drained
I pound canned kidney beans, drained
I pound canned wax beans, drained
I onion, thinly sliced
I green bell pepper, chopped
⅔ cup apple cider vinegar
¼ cup sweetener of your choice (optional)
½ cup olive oil
½ teaspoon freshly ground black pepper

Combine the drained beans in a large bowl with the sliced onion and bell pepper. Mix the vinegar, sweetener, olive oil, and black pepper in a jar; cover and shake well. Pour over the beans and marinate overnight in the refrigerator.

Rice Salad

4 to 6 servings

Use the tofu variation to make a complete meal-in-a-bowl.

I cup brown rice
2 cups water
6 tablespoons olive oil
3 tablespoons apple cider vinegar
Salt and pepper to taste
I tablespoon fresh tarragon
¼ cup minced onion
⅓ cup chopped green pepper or pimiento
½ cup chopped fresh parsley
I cup cooked green peas
I cup cooked asparagus tips
Cherry tomato halves
Green and/or black olives

Simmer the rice in the water until just tender, about 30 minutes. Immediately toss with the olive oil, vinegar, salt, pepper, tarragon, and onion, then set aside to cool. Add the green pepper, parsley, peas, and asparagus tips, and chill. Serve decorated with cherry tomato halves and sliced olives.

Variation: Add ½ pound cubed sautéed tofu.

Couscous Salad

6 cups

This quick-to-make salad is almost a meal in itself.

I cup water
I cup couscous
⅛ teaspoon freshly ground black pepper
3 tablespoons apple cider vinegar
½ teaspoon soy sauce
3 tablespoons olive oil
3 tablespoons sesame seeds
I pound mixed frozen vegetables
½ cup raisins
¼ cup chopped fresh parsley

In a medium saucepan, bring the water to a boil, and stir in the couscous. Cover, remove from the heat, and let stand for about 5 minutes until all the water has been absorbed

Combine the pepper, vinegar, and soy sauce, and set aside.

Sauté the sesame seeds in the olive oil over low heat for a minute or two until they just start to brown. Stir in the frozen vegetables and continue to saute until heated through completely. Remove from the heat. Add the vinegar and soy sauce, and stir in.

Fluff the couscous lightly with a fork. Combine the couscous, vegetables, raisins, and chopped parsley, then toss everything to mix. If you like, you can add a little salt to taste and top with more chopped parsley. Serve warm or chilled.

Homemade Salad Dressing

³⁄₄ cup

I like the clean flavor of canola oil with apple cider vinegar. The sweetener will help you soften the "bite" of this amount of vinegar, if you wish.

½ cup canola oil
⅓ cup apple cider vinegar
¼ teaspoon salt
½ to 1 teaspoon sweetener (optional)

Combine all the ingredients in a jar, shake, and serve. Do not refrigerate.

Try adding all or one of these:

½ clove garlic, crushed (Remove after 24 hours.)
1 teaspoon nutritional yeast
½ teaspoon dry mustard
½ teaspoon paprika
¼ teaspoon black pepper

Quick Gazpacho

4 to 5 servings

Use tomato juice instead of fresh tomatoes for a low-calorie treat that's easy to assemble.

I quart tomato juice

I cucumber, seeded and chopped

I green bell pepper, seeded and chopped

3 stalks celery, chopped

I teaspoon vegetable broth powder

¼ cup apple cider vinegar

I tablespoon vegetarian Worcestershire sauce

I tablespoon chopped fresh parsley

½ teaspoon onion salt

¼ teaspoon freshly ground black pepper

¼ teaspoon garlic powder

Process all the ingredients in several batches in a food processor or blender until smooth. Combine in a large bowl or pitcher, and refrigerate until chilled.

Sweet and Sour Sauce

about 3 cups

¼ cup apple cider vinegar
¾ cup vegetable broth
1 tablespoon ketchup
1 tablespoon soy sauce
1 tablespoon molasses or maple syrup
¼ cup brown sugar or Sucanat
1 (7-ounce) can crushed pineapple
1 tablespoon cornstarch
¼ cup water

Mix all the ingredients in a medium saucepan. Bring to a boil until thickened.

Barbecue Sauce

3 quarts

4 cups vegetable stock
3 (14-ounce) bottles chili sauce
1 teaspoon cayenne pepper
1 teaspoon dry mustard
1½ cups apple cider vinegar
1 clove garlic
4 teaspoons salt
6 tablespoons lemon juice
2 cups olive oil
½ cup flour
½ cup cold water

Combine all the ingredients except the flour and cold water. Cook slowly about 30 minutes. Whisk together the flour and cold water, and stir into the sauce to thicken.

Zesty Mustard

about 3 cups

If you've never made your own mustard before, try this simple recipe. You can experiment with adding chopped fresh herbs and crushed garlic, if you like.

1 cup apple cider vinegar
1 cup dry mustard
2 eggs, beaten
½ cup sugar
Pinch of salt

Combine the vinegar and mustard in a glass bowl; cover, and let stand overnight. Pour into a medium saucepan, and stir in the remaining ingredients. Bring to a slow boil, stirring constantly. Cook until thick, then cool and refrigerate. Keeps for about 4 weeks.

Canning with

Red Pepper Jam

about 14 half-pints

12 large red bell peppers
1 tablespoon salt
3 cups sugar
2 cups apple cider vinegar

Wash the peppers, remove the seeds, and cut into quarters. Mince finely in a food processor. Sprinkle with the salt and let stand for 4 hours. Drain the pepper mixture and add the sugar and vinegar. Cook over moderate heat until thick, about 1 hour. Pour into hot, sterilized half-pint jars, and seal with sterilized canning lids.

Apple Cider Vinegar

Dill Pickles

Brine per quart of cucumbers:
1 teaspoon mustard seed
1 cup apple cider vinegar
2 cups water
1 tablespoon coarse salt

1 teaspoon dill seed or 3 heads fresh dill per quart

Start with cucumbers 3 to 4 inches in length. Scrub them well and pack into hot, sterilized canning jars. Add either the dill seed or heads of fresh dill. Make up enough brine for the number of quarts you're canning, and bring to a boil. Immediately ladle the brine over the cucumbers, filling the jars to within ½ inch of the top of the rim. Top with sterilized caps and rings, and seal tightly. Cool away from drafts.

Green Tomato Mincemeat

10 pints

This is a great vegetarian substitute for traditional mincemeat and makes good use of any green tomatoes you may have at the end of gardening season. It's perfect for pies and in a decorated canning jar becomes a festive homemade gift.

  3 pounds green tomatoes (about 6 cups)
  1½ teaspoons salt
  3½ pounds apples (about 7 cups)
  2 pounds brown sugar
  2 pounds raisins
  2½ tablespoons cinnamon
  1 teaspoon ground cloves
  1½ teaspoons nutmeg
  1 tablespoon grated lemon rind
  3 tablespoons lemon juice
  1¼ cups apple cider vinegar

Mince the tomatoes and grind them in a food processor. Add the salt and let this mixture stand for 1 hour. Drain the tomatoes and add enough water to cover. Bring to a boil and cook for 5 minutes; drain again and set aside. Pare, core, and chop the apples very fine. Place in a large, heavy-bottomed saucepan, and add the tomatoes and remaining ingredients. Mix thoroughly. Bring to a boil, reduce the heat, and simmer gently for 1 hour. Stir frequently. Ladle into 10 hot, sterilized pint canning jars, and seal with sterilized canning lids.

To make a pie with this, preheat the oven to 425°F. Fill an 8-inch pie crust with some of the cooled mixture, and cover with a top crust. Prick the top or cut slits to allow steam to escape. Bake for 15 minutes, then reduce the heat to 375°F and continue baking for 35 minutes.

Pickled Apples

7 pints

These make a delicious accompaniment to winter meals.

4 cups apple cider vinegar
2 cups water
6 cups sugar
2 tablespoons whole cloves
4 cinnamon sticks, broken into bits
8 pounds small apples, cored and peeled

Combine the vinegar, water, and sugar in a large stock pot. Wrap the cloves and cinnamon sticks in cheesecloth, or place them in a stainless steel tea strainer. (Do not use aluminum.) Boil until the sugar has dissolved, add the whole apples, and simmer until tender, about 20 to 30 minutes. Remove the pot from the heat, and let sit for 12 to 18 hours so the flavors will meld.

Pack the apples in 7 sterilized pint jars. Remove the spices from the syrup, bring the syrup back to a boil, and ladle into the jars to ⅛ inch from the top. Cover with canning lids and process in enough boiling water to cover for 10 minutes. Remove the jars and cool on a thick towel or wire rack. Be sure the lids have sealed completely before storing.

Just for Fun
Desserts & Candies

Pastry Dough

dough for 2 crusts

2 cups sifted flour
I teaspoon salt
⅔ cups shortening or nondairy butter substitute
2 tablespoons apple cider vinegar
2 tablespoons milk

Combine the flour and salt in a mixing bowl, then cut in the shortening with a pastry blender or two knives until the mixture looks about the size of small peas. Sprinkle over the vinegar, then the milk, and gather up the flour mixture gently until it just holds together. Do not handle any more than you have to. Roll out and use for pie crusts or other pastry.

Cocoa Cake

1 (9-inch) cake

1½ cups flour
1 cup sugar
¼ cup cocoa
1 teaspoon baking soda
½ teaspoon salt
1 tablespoon apple cider vinegar
1 teaspoon vanilla
⅓ cup canola oil
1 cup cold water

Preheat the oven to 350°F. Combine the flour, sugar, cocoa, baking soda, and salt in a medium mixing bowl. Add the vinegar, vanilla, oil, and cold water, and beat until smooth. Pour into a 9-inch square baking pan, and bake for 30 to 35 minutes. Cool before frosting.

Vinegar Pie

1 (8-inch) pie

This is a basic recipe for "transparent" pie that's a Southern regional favorite.

2 egg yolks
2 cups water
½ cup apple cider vinegar
1 tablespoon melted butter
¼ cup flour
1½ cups sugar
½ teaspoon lemon extract
1 (8-inch) unbaked pie crust

Preheat the oven to 450°F. Beat the egg yolks, water, vinegar, and melted butter together. Mix the flour and sugar, and stir into the vinegar mixture. Add the lemon extract and pour into the pie shell. Bake for 10 minutes, then reduce the heat to 350°F and continue to bake for 20 to 30 minutes until a knife inserted in the edge of the pie comes out clean. Cool before serving.

Holiday Pie

1 (8-inch) pie

This variation of traditional vinegar pie is festive enough for the holidays.

2 eggs
½ cup butter or nondairy spread suitable for baking
1 cup sugar
1 teaspoon vanilla
1 teaspoon vinegar
½ cup chopped nuts
½ cup raisins
½ cup coconut
1 (8-inch) unbaked pie crust

Preheat the oven to 325°F. Mix the eggs, butter, and sugar together. Add the vanilla and vinegar, then fold in the nuts, raisins, and coconut. Pour into the unbaked pie crust, and bake for 45 minutes.

Vinegar Candy

2 cups sugar
½ cup apple cider vinegar
2 tablespoons butter

Combine the ingredients in a large, heavy-bottomed saucepan, and cook until the mixture is brittle when dropped in cold water (270°F on a candy thermometer). Pour onto buttered plates. Mark into squares while warm or roll into small balls.

Old-Fashioned Molasses Candy

2 cups brown sugar
1 cup molasses
1 tablespoon butter
1 tablespoon vinegar
⅛ teaspoon baking soda
1 cup chopped pecans or walnuts

Combine the brown sugar, molasses, butter, and vinegar in a large, heavy-bottomed saucepan, and cook until you have a syrup that will form a hard ball when dropped in cold water (265°F on a candy thermometer). Remove the pan from the heat, add the baking soda, and stir well. Stir in the nuts and pour into a buttered pan. Mark into squares as it cools.

Healthy After Dinner Cordial

If you're looking for a more nutritious end to an elegant meal than an alcoholic beverage, try making a delicious fruit and vinegar cordial. Meld the apple flavors in cider vinegar with other fruits to get a beverage with an after-dinner glow that's truly good for you.

Start with any one of a variety of fruits, such as peaches, strawberries, cherries, blueberries, or black raspberries. Sterilize a quart canning jar, and add 1 cup of 1 or more of the fruits listed above. Sprinkle with a tablespoon of sugar or other lightly flavored sweetener, and cover with 2 cups of apple cider vinegar. Top with a canning lid, and let stand in a dark place for about 2 weeks. Strain off the liquid and serve in small cordial glasses.

Bibliography

Antol, Marie Nadine. *The Incredible Secrets of Vinegar.* New York: Avery, 2000.

Balch, James F., M.D. and Phyllis A. Balch. *Prescription for Nutritional Healing.* New York: Avery, 2000.

Bragg, Paul C., and Patricia Bragg. *Apple Cider Vinegar, Miracle Health System.* Santa Barbara: Health Science.

Browning, Frank. *Apples.* New York: North Point Press, 1998.

Davis, Brenda, and Vesanto Melina. *Becoming Vegan.* Summertown, Tenn.: Book Publishing Company, 2000.

Diggs, Lawrence J. *Vinegar.* Lincoln, Neb.:Authors Choice Press, 2000.

Garrison, Robert, Jr., and Elizabeth Somer. *The Nutrition Desk Reference.* New Canaan, Conn.: Keats, 1995.

Haas, Elson M., M.D. *Staying Healthy with Nutrition.* Berkeley: Celestial Arts, 1992.

Hellmiss, Margot. *Natural Healing with Apple Cider Vinegar.* New York: Sterling Publishing, 1998.

Jarvis, D.C.,MD. *Folk Medicine.* New York: Fawcet Crest, 1958.

Mindell, Earl L., with Larry M. Johns. *Amazing Apple Cider Vinegar.* Los Angeles: Keats Publishing, 1999.

Murray, Michael, and Joseph Pizzorno. *Encyclopedia of Natural Medicine.* Roseville, Cal.: Prima Publishing, 1998.

Oberbeil, Klaus. *Lose Weight with Apple Vinegar.* McKinney, Tex.: Magni Group, 1999.

Orey, Cal. *The Healing Powers of Vinegar.* New York: Kensington Books, 2000.

Scott, Cyril, and John Lust. *Cider Vinegar.* Murray Hill, N.Y.: Benedict Lust Publications, 1992.

Index

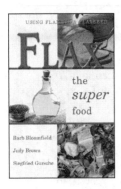 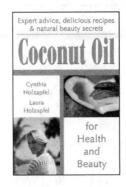 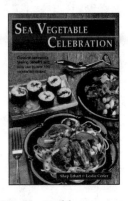
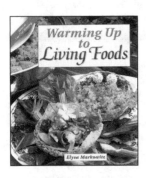 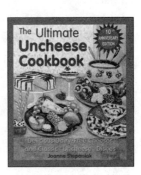 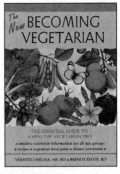